PCOS Polycystic Ovary Syndrome

Everything You Need to Know About PCOS Treatment and Diet Plans to Lead a Productive Life

*By **Cailin Chase***

Disclaimers

Polycystic Ovary Syndrome

Table of Contents

INTRODUCTION 1

CHAPTER 1: WHAT IS POLYCYSTIC OVARY SYNDROME 10

CHAPTER 2: SIGNS, SYMPTOMS AND THE CAUSES OF PCOS 12

CHAPTER 3: COMPLICATIONS OF POLYCYSTIC OVARY SYNDROME 14

TYPE-2 DIABETES
HIGH LEVEL OF CHOLESTEROL
METABOLIC COMPLICATION
CARDIOVASCULAR DISEASE
HEAVYWEIGHT AND OBESITY
ENDOMETRIAL CANCER

CHAPTER 4: THE RISK FACTORS OF POLYCYSTIC OVARY SYNDROME 18

CHAPTER 5: HOW TO IDENTIFY POLYCYSTIC OVARY SYNDROME............................. 20

ASKING HISTORY
PHYSICAL EXAMINATION
PELVIC EXAMINATION
BLOOD TEST VAGINAL ULTRASOUND

CHAPTER 6: MEDICAL TREATMENTS FOR POLYCYSTIC OVARY SYNDROME 22

CHAPTER 7: AYURVEDIC FOR TREATMENTING POLYCYSTIC OVARY SYNDROME.... 27

AYURVEDIC FOR THE OBESE WOMEN WITH INSULIN RESISTANCE AND UNUSUAL BODY HAIR
PCOS TREATMENT FOR THE LEAN WOMEN.

CHAPTER 8: RECIPES 32

CHAPTER 9: CONCLUSION 42

Introduction

How to live a productive life with Polycystic Ovary Syndrome

Can't lose weight? Do you have coarse, abundance hair all over, chest or back? Do you suffer from hair loss or acne? Are you depressed? Unable to conceive?

Assuming this is the case, you're encountering basic manifestations of PCOS (Polycystic Ovary Syndrome). As terrible as these side effects may be, the alarming thing is whether you don't get some control over this disorder, you have a much higher danger of creating cardiovascular infection and diabetes.

Is there a Polycystic Ovarian Syndrome Cure? One without conventional solution? The answer is just yes. Numerous women who suffer this infection accept that they need to live with it their whole lives. They simply need to smile and bear it. This is not genuine and an all-encompassing way to deal with PCOS will take out every one of your side effects.

The standard treatment is to take contraception pills or different medications. Other than undesirable reactions, there is no pill or medication that will stop or cure PCOS.

Regular solutions for polycystic ovary disorder incorporate concentrating vigorously on the eating routine and the procedure of digestion, taking out toxins from the body by taking after detox methods, enhancing and improving the body's own particular resistance and taking measures to roll out way of life improvements for your wellbeing.

Most foods for PCOS are those which we would ordinarily take up with a sound eating regimen. Attempt to eat sensible portion sizes and this is an area where practical judgment skills ought to prevail. PCOS is more common in overweight women so attempt to practice control. It's a no doubt understood truth that women who eat red meats are more defenseless to PCOS, so stick to white meats and fish and attempt to eat natural meat where possible.

Fresh fruits and vegetables are good nourishments for PCOS, albeit sugary fruits and starchy vegetables ought to be eaten in moderation if you suffer from yeast infection. Leafy green vegetables such as kale and cabbage are great natural remedies for polycystic ovary syndrome and women who eat them all the time have fewer incidences of PCOS.

Despite the fact that the calcium in dairy items is essential for bone thickness, numerous alternative specialists propose that dairy foods for PCOS sufferers are not a smart thought. Calcium from different sources, such as, dark lean verdant vegetables, figs, almonds and tinned salmon with bones.

It is totally vital to comprehend that to totally cure yourself of PCOS, it is imperative to look towards utilizing all-encompassing regular solutions for Polycystic Ovarian Syndrome. "All encompassing" means treating the entire body to guarantee that nature is sound and adjusted and it can't flourish. Utilizing isolated cures, for example, foods for PCOS may issue some symptomatic help yet won't cure the condition totally.

Shockingly, Polycystic Ovary Syndrome is not a makeshift issue. On account of its hereditary roots, you will be inclined to PCOS for whatever is left of your life. Hence, you could wind up taking medications for whatever is left of your life. On the off chance that you would prefer not to do that, what else would you be able to do?

To genuinely deal with PCOS, you have to do three fundamental things: enhance your eating routine, get more work out, and lessen stress. Here are fundamental tips of how you can carry on with a profitable existence with Polycystic Ovary Syndrome.

Enhance your carbs

Keep away from refined starches, for example, white bread, white rice, cakes, sweet, breakfast foods, bagels, and other refined grain items. These are "terrible carbs" that make insulin resistance. Insulin resistance is thought to be an essential driver of polycystic ovary disorder.

Refined, made foods by and large have a tendency to bring about you to put on weight, particularly around your center. Better carb decisions are fresh vegetables, fresh fruits, and some whole legumes.

Expand protein

Numerous PCOS women devour a lot of refined carb and insufficient protein. Superb protein helps you to keep your hormones standardized. The best protein sources are fish, poultry, eggs, wild game and amazingly lean meat.

Change your fats.

Some fats and oils aggravate your PCOS side effects while others enhance them. In overabundance, general store vegetables oils, for example, corn oil or man-made fats, for example, "trans-fats" can bring about cells to not work appropriately. Soaked fats found in greasy meats and some dairy items are likewise undesirable. Better decisions incorporate virgin olive oil, flax oil, cod liver oil, and fish oil.

Eat more veggies

A standout amongst the most vital things you can do is to eat all the more vegetables. Attempt to have no less than five vegetable servings a day. Eating a huge amount and assortment of fresh, whole vegetables is a foundation of self-improvement treatment for the numerous wellbeing issues connected with polycystic ovary syndrome.

Control your meal bits

Americans expend unreasonably extensive dinner bits. The more you are served, the more you will eat. Trim the measure of your meal servings. Eat gradually and appreciate a meal. Sit tight for 20 minutes. On the off chance that you are still ravenous, then you can about-face for another part.

Have serving of salad or soup at the start of some meals

Medicinal studies have demonstrated that eating an enormous serving of salad at the start of meals will bring about less aggregate calories eaten at the meal. Soup is another amazing food to help you feel full without expending an excess of calories. Having soup or salad with a meal will make you eat less calories and enhance your capacity to get fitter. What's more, bear in mind, less calories will help you shed pounds and enhance your fruitfulness.

Exercise daily

We frequently feel that we're excessively occupied or hurried, making it impossible to work out. Be that as it may, not practicing is an extravagance you can't manage. PCOS women specifically must practice more than the normal individual. Customary exercises have been demonstrated to enhance polycystic ovary disorder and enhance fruitfulness.

As a minimum, attempt to walk or do other exercises for no less than 30 minutes a day. More is better. Attempt an assortment of activity. Case in point, you may exchange high-impact exercise with weight lifting.

Control stress

Incessant anxiety from any source - your occupation, your life partner, your family, your funds - bothers your hormone adjust, and makes you put on weight around your midsection. Do what you can to enhance any circumstance that is persistently distressing for you. You can likewise deal with changing your state of mind towards a circumstance you see as distressing. Moreover, make certain to require some serious energy for unwinding and relaxing sleep.

Join or form a PCOS support group.

Isolation is not useful. Find other women who are experiencing the same thing you are and communicate now and again to give each other backing and consolidation.

Counsel with a learned health proficient

PCOS is a complex infection that is difficult to treat. Find at least one doctor who fully understands what PCOS is and has some innovative ways of treating it.

Unwind

Managing weight issues or experiencing issues conceiving, PCOS can take a toll on your enthusiastic prosperity. Require some investment out to unwind and appreciate doing something you haven't done in a while. It can have a huge effect by the way you feel within.

Seek help if you are depressed

PCOS can make you feel down, particularly given the huge number of physical and passionate difficulties that can grow as an aftereffect of this infection. In the event that you are feeling quite miserable and can't shake the inclination of helplessness connected with the condition, get help.

Evade stimulants

Coffee and different stimulants cause increments in insulin generation which have a negative effect on ladies with PCOS. On the off chance that you are not kidding about controlling your insulin levels, you truly need to consider your stimulants.

All in all, eating the wrong foods and living a sedentary and stress-filled life will delay or prevent your return to good health. If you follow these tips, you'll be amazed at how much control you have over PCOS and infertility.

All the females with the polycystic ovary ailment may not confront the trouble of getting to be pregnant just those suffering from anovulation may confront the issue. Patients with the issue of anovulation may be treated with clomiphene citrate and FSH infusions. The patients who neglect to give positive results with clomiphene and FSH medications are treated with assisted conceptive innovation technology like controlled ovarian hyperstimulation with follicle invigorating hormone (FSH) infusions took after by in vitro treatment (IVF). Surgery is for the most part not performed in the event of the polycystic ovary but rather a laparoscopic method known as ovarian boring is by and large completed. Hirsutism can be dealt with by utilizing a compelling standard prophylactic pill. The key element of the prophylactic pills is cyproterone acetic acid derivation which is a progestogen. This compound is against androgenic in real life and hinders the movement of male hormones that are in charge of skin break out and undesirable hair development on face and over body. Different medications that convey hostile to androgen impacts incorporate flutamide and spironolactone that can successfully diminish hirsutism. Spironolactone is the most normally utilized medication as a part of the United States.

Menstrual issues can be managed by the utilization of prophylactic pills yet these medications can bring about extra issues if proceeded for quite a while. Two inositol isomers to be specific D-chiro-inositol and myo-inositol have given promising results against this disorder.

Women experiencing polycystic ovary disorder are at the danger of getting influenced with endometrial hyperplasia and endometrial tumor. These clinical indications may manifest because of over amassing of the uterine coating and unlucky deficiency of progesterone which is in charge of the delayed incitement of the uterine cells by estrogen. These manifestations set a positive foundation for the presence of other wellbeing issues like weight, hyperinsulinemia, hyperandrogenism, type 2 diabetes and insulin resistance. A study led in 2010 spotlighted that the ladies experiencing polycystic ovary infection are at a hoisted danger of getting influenced with sort 2 diabetes and insulin resistance. Hypertension, despondency or depression with tension, premature delivery, unreasonable weight increase, cardiovascular illness, acanthosis nigricans, autoimmune thyroiditis are other risks associated with this syndrome.

CHAPTER 1

What Is Polycystic Ovary Syndrome?

Polycystic ovary syndrome (PCOS) is also known as Stein-Leventhal syndrome. It is believed that approximately 5%-10% of women have this condition. It is also the main cause of infertility.

Women with PCOS have a moderate number of small cysts in their ovaries, hence the name poly (many) cystic ovary syndrome.

While the cause of PCOS is unknown, there have been some advances in theories. It is thought that genetics plays a large role in PCOS, therefore, if a mother had PCOS, it is a likely that her daughter will have it. Environmental factors are also thought to be responsible for PCOS.

PCOS is not easy to diagnose. The healthcare provider will take into consideration all signs and symptoms that a woman is exhibiting and analyzes the results from diagnostic (medical) tests.

PCOS is not more common with any particular ethnicity. Unfortunately, many women may not even know that they have PCOS until they are having difficulty in conceiving a child.

Polycystic ovary syndrome (PCOS) is a health problem that can affect a woman's:

- Menstrual cycle
- Ability to have children
- Hormones

- Heart

- Blood vessels

- Appearance

With PCOS, women typically have:

- High levels of androgens. These are sometimes called male hormones, though females also make them.

- Missed or irregular periods (monthly bleeding)

- Many small cysts (fluid-filled sacs) in their ovaries

CHAPTER 2

Signs and Symptoms of PCOS

Polycystic ovary syndrome can often begin early in a woman's life, sometimes as early as when a woman has her first period. PCOS may also happen later in life in the reproductive years.

A hormone that the body produces called insulin may also be linked to PCOS. Insulin is responsible for converting starches, sugar and other foods into a usable form of energy for the body to use or store for later. In PCOS, there is too much insulin in the body and it cannot be used appropriately. This excess in insulin can increase the production of androgens. Androgens is a male hormone that exists in smaller levels in females. When there is an increased amount of androgens, we will start to see increased body hair and possible male pattern baldness.

Below are some signs and symptoms of PCOS:

- Infertility (not able to get pregnant) because of not ovulating. In fact, PCOS is the most common cause of female infertility.

- Infrequent, absent, and/or irregular menstrual periods

- Hirsutism - Increased hair growth on the face, chest, stomach, back, thumbs, or toes

- Cysts on the ovaries

- Acne, oily skin, or dandruff

- Weight gain or obesity, usually with extra weight around the waist

- Male-pattern baldness or thinning hair

- Patches of skin on the neck, arms, breasts, or thighs that are thick and dark brown or black

- Skin tags - Excess flaps of skin in the armpits or neck area

- Pelvic pain

- Anxiety or Depression

- Sleep Apnea - When breathing stops for short periods of time while asleep

CHAPTER 3

Complications of PCOS

There can be a variety of complications from PCOS. Many of these complication may be observed if obesity is seen:

Irregular menstrual cycle and infertility: A woman's eggs are located in the ovaries. In the ovaries are follicles, which are tiny fluid filled sacs. As the egg matures the follicle will open and release the egg where it will travel down the fallopian tube to the uterus for fertilization. This also known as the process of ovulation.

However, in PCOS, the ovary will not make enough hormone for the egg to mature. The follicles start to grow and collect fluid, but the egg is not released so ovulation does not occur. As a result a hormone called progesterone will not be made. If progesterone is not made, the menstrual cycle will become irregular or absent.

Pregnancy and PCOS: While it is possible to become pregnant with PCOS, there appears to be a higher incidence of:

- Miscarriage
- Still born baby
- Miscarriage
- Gestational diabetes
- Pregnancy-induced high blood pressure (preeclampsia)
- Premature delivery

Babies born to women with PCOS have a higher risk of spending time in a neonatal intensive care unit or of dying before, during, or shortly after birth. Most of the time, these problems occur in multiple-birth babies (twins, triplets).

Type-2 diabetes: Women who are suffering from polycystic ovary syndrome can have type 2 diabetes after few years. This theory is applicable to all the women who have PCOS, but it depends on the production of insulin. Difficulties in insulin production can develop type-2 diabetes in a PCOS patient. About 50 percent of women found with having type-2 diabetes during diagnosis. Type-2 diabetes happens due to an imbalance of insulin. The risk of having type-2 diabetes increases by the following factors;

• Overweight.

• The resistance of insulin.

High cholesterol: High level of testosterone hormone triggers the cholesterol level in your blood. As a result you can have heart disease and even a heart attack. High level of cholesterol "LDL" (bad level for health) can also cause blockages in the heart. Women with the polycystic ovary syndrome can also have the low level of cholesterol "HDL" (good level of cholesterol for health) and raise triglycerides (another form of fat in your blood).

Metabolic complications: Metabolic complications are the signs and symptoms that include; abdominal pain, high blood pressure, unusual cholesterol level and resistance of insulin. This complexity can lead to heart disease.

Cardiovascular disease: Women who have PCOS, can develop cardiovascular disease. There are different factors that can trigger a cardiovascular disease. Such as;

• Excess fat and cholesterol in the blood.

• High level of bad cholesterol and reduced lipoprotein cholesterol.

• The increasing level of inflammatory proteins which can affect the usual function of the blood vessels and raise insulin resistance.

• High blood pressure.

Obesity: Polycystic ovary syndrome can occur in women of any weight. Different researchers say that, about 75 percent of women with polycystic ovary syndrome are overweight.

Gaining weight especially having a large amount of abdominal fat are associated with:

• An increasing risk of insulin resistance.

• Having problems with infertility.

• An increasing risk of having type-2 diabetes.

• An increasing risk of cardiovascular disease. For an example; high blood pressure, stroke and heart block.

Endometrial cancer: PCOS carries an additional risk of endometrial cancer. Due to the absence of ovulation, estrogen is produced, but, progesterone is not. Progesterone is responsible for the lining of the uterus (endometrium) to shed every month. Without progesterone, the endometrium becomes thickened causing heavy and/or irregular bleeding. As time passes, endometrial hyperplasia and endometrial cancer can occur.

The best way to prevent complications from PCOS that you can do is:

- Stop smoking

- Eat a balanced diet

- Exercise

As you already know, the three preventative actions above, can make a big difference in the severity of complications that comes with PCOS.

CHAPTER 4

The Risk Factors for Polycystic Ovary Syndrome

Women with PCOS have greater chances of developing several serious health conditions, including life-threatening diseases. Recent studies found that:

- Women with PCOS are at greater risk of having high blood pressure.

- Women with PCOS have high levels of LDL (bad) cholesterol and low levels of HDL (good) cholesterol.

- More than 50 percent of women with PCOS will have diabetes or pre-diabetes (impaired glucose tolerance) before the age of 40.

- The risk of heart attack is 4 to 7 times higher in women with PCOS than women of the same age without PCOS.

- Women with PCOS can develop sleep apnea. This is when breathing stops for short periods of time during sleep.

- Women with PCOS may also develop anxiety and depression. It is important to talk to your doctor about treatment for these mental health conditions.

Women with PCOS are also at risk for endometrial cancer. Irregular menstrual periods and the lack of ovulation cause women to produce the hormone estrogen, but not the hormone progesterone. Progesterone causes the endometrium (lining of the womb) to shed each month as a menstrual period. Without progesterone, the endometrium becomes thick, which can cause heavy or irregular bleeding. Over time, this can lead to endometrial hyperplasia, when the lining grows too much, and cancer.

When the women with polycystic ovary syndrome give birth of a baby, then there can be a terrible condition. The baby may send along with the mother into an intensive care unit. This complication happens during delivery or after the short time birth. These problems occur with multiple-fetus. That means this can happen mostly in case of giving birth twins and triplets. Different researchers are experimenting in this case to find out whether metformin (a diabetes reducing medicine) can help to prevent or lower the chances of having these issues during pregnancy. Metformin is used to lower down the male hormone (testosterone) levels and barricades the weight gain for women. Especially, who get obsessed when they get pregnant.

Metformin is a "B category" drug for the pregnant women approved by the FDA. It does not cause any major birth defects or other problems during pregnancy. But, there are few studies for the use of metformin for the pregnant women to confirm its safety. You should ask your doctor about taking metformin, if you are pregnant or are willing to become pregnant. Metformin is also passed for breastfeeding. You must discuss with your doctor about the use of metformin, if you are a nursing mother.

CHAPTER 5

How to Identify Polycystic Ovary Syndrome

Diagnosis is generally made by "exclusion", this means that the healthcare provider will need to consider all other possible illnesses that can cause similar signs and symptoms, including but not limited to hypothyroidism and other hormonal pathologies or illnesses. The following test may be used to help come up with a diagnosis of PCOS:

- **History and Physical**- Your doctor will ask about your menstrual periods, weight changes, and other symptoms. Your doctor will want to measure your blood pressure, body mass index (BMI), and waist size. He or she also will check the areas of increased hair growth. You should try to allow the natural hair to grow for a few days before the visit.

- **Pelvic Examination**- Your doctor might want to check to see if your ovaries are enlarged or swollen by the increased number of small cysts.

- **Transvaginal Ultrasound**- This is a painless exam that will allow the healthcare provider to visualize the ovaries and the uterus. Your doctor may perform a test that uses sound waves to take pictures of the pelvic area. It might be used to examine your ovaries for cysts and check the endometrium (lining of the womb). This lining may become thicker if your periods are not regular.

- **Blood Tests**- Your doctor may check the androgen hormone and glucose (sugar) levels in your blood.

CHAPTER 6

Medical Treatments for PCOS

Types of medical treatment: You should talk to your physician you think that you may be suffering from polycystic ovary syndrome. While there is no cure for the polycystic ovary syndrome. Different medical techniques and lifestyle modifications are the best options to treat the polycystic ovary syndrome.

Some of the treatments are given below:

Contraceptive pills or birth control pills:

- Helps to modify the unusual period cycle.

- Reduces testosterone hormone (male hormone).

- This can possibly reduce problems with acne.

- Doctors may suggest birth control pills to help with ovulation and conception.

Metformin: This medication has been found helpful to slow or mitigate the incidence of polycystic ovary syndrome. Metformin works like insulin. Metformin Modifies the sugar level in the blood and reduces the testosterone hormone. It is used to treat the other problems like unusual hair growth and weight gain. This medication can also assist with the ovulation process.

Fertility Medications: Irregular ovulation is usually found in women who are suffering from polycystic ovary syndrome. Different researchers have shown that about 70% of women diagnosed with polycystic ovary syndrome have infertility.

Treatments for infertility:

- **Clomid** – a medication to help with the ovulation cycle.

- **Metformin** - This medication has been found helpful to slow or mitigate the incidence of polycystic ovary syndrome. Metformin works like insulin. Metformin Modifies the sugar level in the blood and reduces the testosterone hormone. It is used to treat the other problems like unusual hair growth and weight gain. This medication can also assist with the ovulation process.

- **Letrozole:** This is an oral medication. Letrozole that works like Clomid. Letrozole may also be the first choice to stimulate the ovulation process. This medication can also be suggested by your practitioner, but the dosage and treatment policy may vary depending on your physician.

- **Gonadotropins:** This medicine is used in a short form. Gonadotropin is used to stimulate the ovary to produce enough follicles. This medication should also be suggested by your doctor, but dosage and treatment instruction may vary depending on your doctor.

- **In vitro fertilization or IVF** – Best chance in becoming pregnant. This option is very expensive.

Surgery for the PCOS

Ovarian Drilling: This is a process when a doctor makes a very tiny hole above or below the surface of the navel and pushes a small tool that acts like a telescope into the abdomen. This process is also known as a laparoscopy (medical surgery). After that, the doctor pinches the ovary with a small needle by carrying an electric current. This electricity helps to destroy a small portion of the ovary. This surgical process may lower the level of male hormone (testosterone hormone) and help with ovulation system. Sometimes it may carry a risk of having a scar tissue on the surface of the ovary. The benefits of this surgery may only last for a few months. There are both benefits and risk of this surgery. You should ask your doctor if you feel any discomfort after this surgery. Your doctor will do an assessment based on the complaint and decide on the treatment if necessary.

Oophorectomy: Your ovaries contain eggs that produce hormones to ease your menstrual or period cycle. An oophorectomy is a surgical procedure where your surgeon may remove one or both ovaries. The method will call as a Bilateral Oophorectomy when both ovaries are removed. This surgery is typically performed with other procedures like a hysterectomy surgery. Your doctor can suggest this surgery if it is the right treatment for your symptoms.

Hysterectomy: At the time of hysterectomy surgery, a surgeon removes the uterus and cervix of women. Sometimes your doctor may choose to remove the uterus only. If your doctor only removes the uterus, then it will call a partial hysterectomy surgery. You should discuss the procedure and the further complications with your doctor.

Medication for unusual hair growth or increasing testosterone hormone:

Vaniqa: This is a cream that helps to reduce the extra facial hair. The risks, dosage and side effects of this medication should be discussed with your doctor. If you face any allergy or facial complication, then you must visit your doctor chamber immediately.

Aldactone: It is used to block the androgens or male hormones. You should discuss the risks, dosage and side effects with your doctor or practitioner.

Modification of your lifestyle

You should know about the nutrition facts. You should find someone who is specialized in PCOS or Diabetes and can give you particular advice regarding nutrition.

- You must know about the nutrition label
- You must broadly learn about "Glycemic Index (GI and Glycemic Load (GL))".
- You should try to restore your diet.
- You should eat and learn about the meal that is full of nutrition.

- You can perform an exercise for both cardiovascular and weight loss. You should maintain the proper training method that recommended by your doctor or trainer.
- You can also do meditation to reduce your anxiety, Breathing problem, Depression, and Stress.
- You should avoid smoking, if you are diagnosed with polycystic ovary syndrome.
- You should avoid processed foods and foods with highly added sugar.
- You should add many whole-grain foods, fruit, deep green vegetable and meat to your everyday meal plan.

Treatments for weight loss

Medically approved weight loss programs: The Common medical research says that, a lower body weight can reduce the risk factors for disease.

Bariatric surgery: In most cases, this surgical treatment may help the women who are suffering from Obese. You must visit your health care professional to discuss if which surgical process is suitable for you.

Other treatments:

- Laser hair removal surgery.
- Medically approved hormonal treatments.
- Alternative methods.
- Different vitamins and minerals supplement.

CHAPTER 7

Different Ayurvedic medicines for the treatments of polycystic ovary syndrome.

Ayurvedic medicine for polycystic ovary syndrome

Shatavari (Asparagus recess): Shatavari helps a pregnant woman with PCOS to produce the normal development of ovarian follicles. Shatavari helps to regulate the unusual menstrual cycle and restore the female reproductive system. Shatavari is also helpful with the hyperinsulinemia. Shatavari can also reduce hyperinsulinemia (high level of insulin) because of its phytoestrogen (a kind of natural plant-based estrogen).

Guduchi (Tinospora Cordifolia): Guduchi is one of the most powerful anti- inflammatory herbal medicines. A chronic inflammation in tissues is the primary cause of insulin imbalance and ovarian cysts. Guduchi helps a woman with PCOS restoring all the body tissues and boost up the metabolic system naturally. This herb also helps to lower down the insulin resistance of a woman with polycystic ovary syndrome.

Shatapushpa (Foeniculum vulgare): The fennel seed is famous as Shatapushpa. In Sanskrit book, Shatapushpa is described as an excellent supplement for the treatment of polycystic ovary syndrome. This herb is rich in phytoestrogens. Phytoestrogens (a natural estrogen) helps in reducing the insulin resistance level and in lower down the inflammation in polycystic ovary syndrome. Phytoestrogens also known as a helping herb that reduces the cellular imbalance. A cellular imbalance may lead you to metabolic disturbances in PCOS.

Triphala: A mixture of three fruits- Amalaki (Emblica Officinalis), Haritaki (Terminalia nebula) and Bibhitaki (Terminalia bellerica) are known as Triphala. Triphala is the most popular Ayurvedic treatments containing classical formulations. It has a rich source of vitamin C (a powerful natural antioxidant) that helps to reduce the swelling by producing free radicals. Triphala associates in cleansing and detoxifying your system. It is the best herb from any other Ayurvedic medicines that will help you to cure polycystic ovary syndrome.

Aloe Vera- Kumari (Aloe barb adenosis): Aloe Vera is another Ayurvedic herb that is extremely beneficial to treat the patient with PCOS. It helps to regularize the period cycles, promotes a usual menstruation and normalizes the hormonal imbalance of ovary.

Ashwagandha roots: Ashwagandha is also a well-known herbal supplement. It is an extensive application in traditional Indian and Ayurvedic medicine. Ashwagandha is always highly prized for its importance and treatment for infertility. Ashwagandha root is highly prescribed in Ayurveda to treat the PCOD patient. An exclusive paste made from the particular amount of Ashwagandha roots and Arjun bark heavily prescribed for PCOD patients.

Sesame seeds: For making this herb, first boil 5 grams of black sesame seeds in 100 ml of water. Then filter the boiling water and add organic jaggery. You can drink it two times a day on empty stomach. You can get twice benefits if you drink the water in the morning. This simple remedy can be helpful to reconstruct your period cycle and stomach problem.

Some Ayurvedic treating methods are described below

Ayurvedic Treatment for the obese woman with insulin resistance and unusual body hair.

Phase 1: Preparatory Phase.

- Selected Ayurvedic medicine and diet should include with Carminative, Digestive and moderate laxative qualities.
- The medicine and the diet should have the quality to reduce body weight and cholesterol.
- Must have the power to reduce the glucose level in the blood. It will lower down your cravings, tiredness and barricades the excess hair growth.

Phase 2: Detoxification or purification (Panchakarma).

A detoxification process should contain an internal location, sweating, therapeutic purgation and Vashti's.

Vashti must include vatha reducing, pitha pacifying and weight reducing qualities. This vasthi alone can give you a very fast result.

Utharavasthi medicines must contain some potentials to reach the uterus, then to the fallopian tube and finally to ovaries. This helps for the rapture or shrinks the follicles.

Phase 3: Internal medication

An internal medication is used to balance the ratio of LH / FSH and reconstruct the menstruation cycle and system.

Phase 4: Internal medicine – for long-term sustained benefits

Rasayana and fertility medications: Rasayana is a group of herbal medicine remedies. The antioxidant properties of Rasayana are used in Ayurveda treatment to restore health, protect you against disease, and promote longevity.

PCOS Treatment for Lean Women

As per Ayurvedic dosha view for the treatment of the lean women, Vata dosha develops your system slowly but Kapha dosha grows only in the local area and around the pelvic area.

Phase 1: Pre-Treatment or preparatory phase

You can Correct Agni, Aparna Vayu and blood glucose level by a good nutrient plan and carminative medicines.

Selection of ayurvedic medicines should contain the facts written below:

- Vata pacifying nature is the mandatory facts of these medicines.
- These medicines should have a super digestive formula.

- Natural mild-laxative formula.

- These medicines should contain a nourishing quality.

- Hormone balancing capability.

Phase 2: Ayurveda detoxification or purification (Pancha karma)

- Internal operation with medicated ghee (they have Vata pacifying formula and hormones balancing qualities).

- Sweating and therapeutic purgation may remove toxins from your body and destroys ama that blocks Aparna Vayu.

- Vasthi with vatha Samana and nourishing medicines.

- Utharavathi is for shrinking or bursting the cyst in the ovary.

Phase 3: Internal Medication

Internal medicines can rebuild LH/FSH ratio and correct your menstrual cycle.

Phase 4: Internal medicines – long term benefits

Rasayana and fertility medication.

Recipes

Breakfast

Dairy free Blueberry Muesli

Serves 4

Ingredients:

1 1/2 cups rolled oats
1/2 cup walnuts, chopped
1/2 cup dried apples, chopped
2 tsp ground cinnamon
2 cups blueberries (preferably wild)
3 tbsp brown sugar
Apple juice, to serve

Directions:

Preheat oven to 325°F

Mix oats, sugar, and cinnamon in a bowl. Spread mixture evenly onto a non-stick baking tray.

Toast oat mixture in preheated oven for about 10 minutes, stirring occasionally. Watch mixture very closely when toasting as it can burn very easily.

Remove from oven and let cool. Pour into a large bowl and stir in chopped walnuts and dried apples.

Divide mixture into serving bowls and top with blueberries. Serve with apple juice.

Breakfast

Low Glycemic Raspberry Muffins

Serves 10

Ingredients:

1 1/2 cups whole wheat flour
1/2 cup soy flour
2 tsp baking powder
1/3 cup brown sugar
2 tsp cinnamon
2 egg whites
1 cup soy milk
2 Tbsp canola oil
1 cup raspberries

Directions:

Preheat oven to 375°F

Combine dry ingredients in a large bowl. Whisk together egg whites, soy milk, and canola oil in a separate bowl.

Add wet ingredients to dry ingredients and mix until just blended (do not over-mix). Fold in raspberries.

Fill 12 paper muffin cups with batter (about two thirds full). Bake until a tester toothpick comes out clean, about 15-20 minutes.

Breakfast

Weight Loss Muffins

Serves 12

Ingredients:

1 cup rolled oats, soaked in 1 cup skim milk for 1-2 hours
1/2 cup unsweetened applesauce
2 egg whites
1 cup skim milk
1 cup whole wheat flour
1/2 cup brown sugar
1 tsp baking powder
1/2 tsp baking soda
1/2 tsp salt
1 tsp cinnamon
1 cup blueberries

Directions:

Preheat oven to 400 degrees F

Beat together egg whites, oat-milk mixture, and applesauce. Combine dry ingredients in a separate bowl.

Add liquid ingredients to dry ingredients and mix until just combined (do not over-mix). Fold in blueberries.

Fill 12 paper muffin cups with batter (about two thirds full). Bake for 20 minutes or until done.

Main Dishes

Nettle Pesto with Whole-wheat Pasta

<u>Ingredients</u>

2 cups young nettle leaves, blanched
4 garlic cloves, peeled
1/3 cup walnuts, chopped
1/3 cup Parmesan cheese, grated
1/3 cup extra-virgin olive oil
12 oz dried whole-wheat pasta

<u>Directions</u>

Combine nettle leaves, garlic, and walnuts in a food processor. Process while gradually adding olive oil until you reach desired consistency. Stir in grated Parmesan cheese.

Cook pasta according to package directions to al dente.

Drain pasta, put back in the pot, and stir in nettle pesto.

Transfer onto serving plates and garnish as desired.

Main Dishes

Onion & Apple Soup

Ingredients

1 Tbsp canola oil
2 medium yellow onions, sliced
1 small leek, chopped
1/2 Tbsp fresh rosemary, chopped
1/2 Tbsp fresh thyme
3 organic apples, cut into small dices
6 cups fat-free, low-sodium vegetable broth

Directions

Heat the oil in a medium saucepan over medium heat. Add the onions and sauté until golden.

Pour in the broth and bring to the boil over medium-high heat. Add the apples, and reduce the heat to medium-low. Simmer for 10 minutes.

Main DIshes

Chicken Salad with Pine Nuts & Dried Cranberries

Ingredients

1 3/4 oz skinless chicken breasts, cooked and sliced
1/2 medium red onion, thinly sliced
1/2 cucumber, halved lengthwise, sliced
1/4 cup fresh basil, coarsely chopped
1/2 cup dried cranberries
10 oz romaine lettuce, washed and torn
3 Tbsp balsamic vinegar
1 Tbsp canola oil
1 Tbsp honey
1 small garlic clove, minced
Salt, to taste
Freshly ground black pepper, to taste
1/4 cup pine nuts

Directions:

Combine first six ingredients in a large bowl. In a small bowl, whisk together vinegar, canola oil, honey, and minced garlic, salt, and pepper. Drizzle over salad mixture and toss gently.

Sprinkle with pine nuts. Chill before serving.

Barley & Broccoli Soup

Ingredients

1/4 cup yellow onion, chopped
1 small carrot, peeled and diced
1 rib organic celery, finely chopped
1 tbsp extra virgin olive oil
4 cups small, organic broccoli florets
1/2 cup pearled barley, cooked
5 cups vegetable broth
1 can (14 1/2 oz) stewed tomatoes
4 cloves garlic, minced
1/4 tsp dried marjoram
1 tsp thyme
Salt and pepper, to taste

Directions

In a stock pot, cook onion in olive oil over medium heat for 4-5 minutes until soft.

Add vegetable broth and bring to a boil. Reduce to a simmer and add celery and carrots along with broccoli florets. Cover and let simmer until carrots and broccoli florets are tender.

Add cooked barley, canned tomatoes, garlic, marjoram, and thyme. Let simmer another minute or two.

Season with salt and pepper. Serve warm

Main Dishes

Eggs & Shrimp on Romaine

Ingredients

2 cups shrimp, cooked, peeled and chilled
1/2 cup cherry tomatoes, halved
1/3 cup extra light mayonnaise
1/4 cup chili sauce
3 Tbsp lemon juice
Romaine lettuce
3 hard-boiled eggs, halved
2 cups watercress, trimmed

Directions

Whisk together mayonnaise, chili sauce, and lemon juice in a small bowl. Cover and refrigerate for at least 30 minutes.

In a large bowl, combine shrimp, and cherry tomatoes. Pour in chili mayonnaise dressing and toss lightly.

Deserts

Whole Wheat Brownies

Ingredients

3 tbsp low-sodium butter
1/2 cup brown rice syrup
10 tbsp dark cocoa powder, unsweetened
1 tsp vanilla
2 eggs
1/2 cup whole wheat flour
1/2 cup pecans, chopped

Directions

In a medium saucepan, melt butter over low heat. Stir in brown rice syrup, and whisk in cocoa powder. Continue whisking until well blended.

Remove from heat and blend in eggs.

Add in vanilla, whole wheat flour, and pecans, and stir well.

Lightly grease 8x8-inch baking pan and pour in batter. Bake for 30 minutes or until a toothpick comes out clean

Cool & cut into squares.

Quinoa Crepes with Applesauce

Serves 10-12

Ingredients

1 1/2 quinoa flour
1/2 cup tapioca flour
1 tsp baking soda
1 tsp cinnamon
2 cup carbonated water
3 tbsp canola oil
3 cups unswtnd, organic apple sauce
Cinnamon, to taste

Directions

In a medium bowl, mix together quinoa flour, tapioca flour, baking soda, and cinnamon. Add water and oil and whisk until well combined.

Preheat a large nonstick skillet over medium heat. Add a few drops of canola oil.

For first crepe, pour about 1/3 cup of batter into skillet, rotating skillet quickly until bottom is evenly coated. Cook crepe on medium high heat until bottom is light brown. Flip over and briefly cook other side.

Repeat previous step until batter is gone. Serve with apple sauce.

Conclusion

Thank you for reading this full book. I have written all the information about 'polycystic ovary syndrome'. Don't be frustrated about polycystic ovary syndrome. Knowledge can go a long way in treatment and prevention.

www.ingramcontent.com/pod-product-compliance
Lightning Source LLC
Chambersburg PA
CBHW070841290526
45795CB00002B/938